Claudia D. Spies · Benno Rehberg · Stephan A. Schug
Gunnar Jaehnichen · Sarah J. Harper
(Eds.)

Pocket Guide Pain Management

Claudia D. Spies · Benno Rehberg
Stephan A. Schug · Gunnar Jaehnichen
Sarah J. Harper
(Eds.)

Pocket Guide
Pain Management

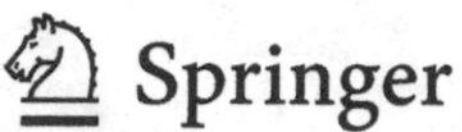

Prof. Dr. med. Claudia D. Spies, Berlin
Dr. med. Benno Rehberg, Berlin
Prof. Stephan A. Schug, MD FANZCA FFPMANZCA, Perth
Dr. med. Gunnar Jaehnichen, Delmenhorst
Dr. Sarah J. Harper, Gloucestershire

ISBN 978-3-540-32996-1 ISBN 978-3-540-32997-8(eBook)

DOI 10.1007/978-3-540-32997-8

Library of Congress Control Number: 2008926229

Cover design: Frido Steinen-Broo, eStudio Calamar, Spain
Production & Typesetting: le-tex publishing services oHG, Leipzig, Germany

Printed on acid-free paper

9 8 7 6 5 4 3 2 1

springer.com

Preface

In the United States about 50 million people suffer from recurrent or chronic pain, and nearly 10% of adults take medication for pain daily. Further, the disease burden of pain is expected to grow, relative to other illnesses and conditions.

Despite the advances in pain medicine, most physicians are not adequately trained to treat chronic or even acute pain. As in other fields of medicine, pain medicine has long been dominated by expert opinion relying on personal expertise, and only recently has a systematic evaluation of treatments in the terms of "evidence-based medicine" been performed.

And also as in other fields of medicine, a lot can be achieved in pain medicine when certain basic diagnostic and therapeutic pathways are followed correctly; more than can be achieved when only a few specialists are able to treat these conditions.

"Standard operating procedures" (SOPs) are supposed to be concise practical aids for clinicians, standardizing treatments, diagnostic pathways and procedures in one of sometimes many possible ways. Although based on the available evidence, they are not evidence-based guidelines and are not supposed to replace such guidelines. On one hand, evidence-based medicine often leaves many options open, since in many cases the available evidence is not sufficient to recommend a specific option. On the other hand, there might be reasons due to clinical practice (e.g. metamizol cannot be used in Scandinavia due to genetic predispositions) that specific options are not left open. In this context, SOPs can guide the clinician to choose an option within the best available evidence in the context of their daily practice.

This book is based on the SOPs of the Charité – Universitätsmedizin Berlin university hospital and medical school in Berlin. These SOPs, local in origin, have gained widespread acceptance in many hospitals throughout Germany after being published as a book. Meanwhile, they have also been adopted by the German Society of Anesthesiologists as part of a countrywide quality management project.

The adaptation of the pain therapy part of these SOPs for an international audience has been accomplished by Professor Stephan A. Schug and his team at the University of Western Australia.

The editors and authors hope that these "SOPs" will replace single expert opinions, and provide more physicians with evidence-based knowledge and options to implement the SOPs in their clinical routine in order to treat pain patients adequately and to improve their clinical outcomes.

August 2008

Claudia D. Spies
Benno Rehberg
Stephan A. Schug
Gunnar Jaehnichen
Sarah J. Harper

Contents

List of Editors

Prof. Dr. med. Claudia D. Spies
Charité, Klinik für Anästhesiologie
und operative Intensivmedizin
Campus Charité Mitte und Campus Virchow Klinikum
Schumannstraße 20–21
10117 Berlin
Germany

Dr. med. Benno Rehberg
Charité, Klinik für Anästhesiologie
und operative Intensivmedizin
Campus Charité Mitte und Campus Virchow Klinikum
Schumannstraße 20–21
10117 Berlin
Germany

Professor Stephan A. Schug, MD FANZCA FFPMANZCA
Professor and Chair of Anaesthesiology
Pharmacology and Anaesthesiology Unit
School of Medicine and Pharmacology
University of Western Australia
& Director of Pain Medicine, Royal Perth Hospital
UWA Anaesthesia
GPO Box X2213
Perth, WA 6847
Australia

Dr. med. Gunnar Jaehnichen
Leitender Oberarzt der Klinik für Anästhesiologie
Palliativmedizin und Schmerztherapie
Wildeshauser Str. 92
27753 Delmenhorst
Germany

Dr. Sarah J. Harper MB ChB FRCA
Consultant in Anaesthesia and Pain Medicine
Gloucestershire Hospitals NHS Foundation Trust
Department of Anaesthesia
Gloucestershire Royal Hospital
Great Western Road
Gloucester GL1 3NN
UK

List of Contributors

Dr. med. Michael Schenk
Gemeinschaftskrankenhaus Havelhöhe gGmbH
Klinik für Anästhesiologie
Kladower Damm 221
14089 Berlin

Dr. med. Eva Hoffmann
DRK-Kliniken Berlin Westend
Spandauer Damm 130
14050 Berlin

Dipl.-Psych. Hilde Urnauer
Ostseestr. 107
10409 Berlin

Dr. med. Tamina Machholz
Asklepios Klinik Birkenwerder
Hubertusstraße 12–22
16547 Birkenwerder

1 General Principles of Pain Management

M. Schenk, E. Hoffmann, H. Urnauer,
S.A. Schug, G. Jaehnichen, S.J. Harper

In Germany an estimated 5 million people (8% of the population) suffer from chronic pain. Worldwide, the prevalence of chronic benign pain ranges between 2% and 40% of the population, depending on the study. In the USA, the rate of disability claims associated with chronic back pain has increased above the rate of population growth by 1,400%. Often these chronic pain patients have been reviewed by many physicians and have tried a variety of different treatments. They often have impaired ability to perform daily activities and have associated psychological disorders and social problems.

A wide range of therapeutic options dealing with both the individual problems and biopsychosocial context of these chronic pain patients is needed. Methods and techniques used in pain therapy are constantly developed and improved. Efficacy must be reappraised frequently, ideally using the results of new multidisciplinary clinical trials or high quality meta-analyses. Physicians and psychologists working in pain therapy should have special training and experience in this field.

Multidisciplinary Approach in Pain Therapy

Treatment of chronic pain in pain clinics needs a multidisciplinary approach, based on the theory that chronification of pain can be caused by somatization as well as by social and psychological factors. For assessment of these factors a multidisciplinary diagnostic evaluation is necessary. To achieve multidisciplinary diagnosis, practitioners of different backgrounds, including physicians and psychologists, perform a first assessment together, study the available information, and set up an individualized therapy plan. This therapy plan may focus more on medical or on psychological treatment strategies depending on the individual case. The overall coordination of the treatment usually lies in the hands of the medical pain specialist.

For optimization of therapeutic success it is important that each member of the team is well-informed about the progress of the pain therapy. This allows constant adjustment of the goals of therapy and appropriate definition of new goals when required. A multidisciplinary pain team usually includes neurologists, specialists in physical therapy and psychosomatic medicine, as well as the anesthetic pain specialist and psychologist.

Multidisciplinary pain meetings, attended by pain physicians, psychologists and general practitioners are of key importance.

1.1 Pain Evaluation

Besides a thorough examination of the patient, pain evaluation is the basis for pain diagnosis and pain therapy. In preparation for the pain evaluation, a pain questionnaire answered by the patient should be evaluated. Worldwide, there are many pain questionnaires for the evaluation of chronic pain available and they should contain some of the following:

- Personal data
- Description of pain (location, character, intensity, development over time)
- Co-morbidity
- Pain development and treatment so far
- Social situation (private situation, situation at work, social status)

Some examples of internationally used pain evaluation tools:

1. PDI (Pain Disability Index): This brief instrument was developed to assess pain-related disability, providing information that complements an assessment of physical impairment. It is a self-report instrument assessing the degree to which chronic pain interferes with various daily activities.

2. MPI/WHYMPI (West Haven-Yale Multidimensional Pain Inventory): This 52-item inventory contains 12 scales divided into 3 parts: 1) interference, support, pain severity, self-control and negative mood; 2) punishing responses, solicitous responses and distracting responses; 3) household chores, outdoor work, activities away from home and social activities. Translations in Dutch, French, Italian, Portuguese, Spanish, Swedish and other languages are available.
3. CPCI (Chronic Pain Coping Inventory): As coping strategies are among the psychosocial factors hypothesized to contribute to the development of chronic musculoskeletal disability, this inventory was developed to assess 8 behavioral coping strategies targeted in multidisciplinary pain treatment (guarding, resting, asking for assistance, task persistence, relaxation, exercise/stretch, coping self-statements and seeking social support). The scales of this instrument can be grouped according to the following coping families: 1) illness focused coping and 2) wellness-focused coping.
4. BDI (Becks Depression Inventory) or HADS (Hospital Anxiety and Depression Scale): HADS might be used as an instrument that is designed to detect the presence and severity of mild degrees of mood disorder, anxiety and depression.

1.2 Documentation of Pain

Documentation systems for chronic pain are important for:
1. Understanding the subjective components of pain
2. Improving communication between the pain therapist and other health care professionals looking after the patient
3. Quality control of pain diagnosis and pain therapy

Pain Diaries

Pain diaries are essential for the evaluation of pain development. Pain diaries are available for different types of pain and usually cover the symptoms of the specific type of pain. The following contents of pain diaries help patients and pain therapists to understand the biopsychosocial factors influencing their pain:

- Pain intensity
- Duration of pain
- General health
- Effects of the pain
- Limitation of activities
- Medication

Evaluation of Pain Severity

For evaluation of subjective pain intensity, three different measuring systems are available in routine clinical practice. With all three measuring systems, patients refer to their pain in relation to a number or diagram. These systems are an important part of pain assessment, pain development and quality control in pain therapy.

Visual Analogue Scale (VAS)

On an unscaled ruler (Fig. 1), patients select a value between pain free (VAS 0) and unbearable pain (VAS 10 or 100). The pain therapist is able to read the corresponding value on the other side of the ruler. This technique is only partially suitable for patients with impaired consciousness.

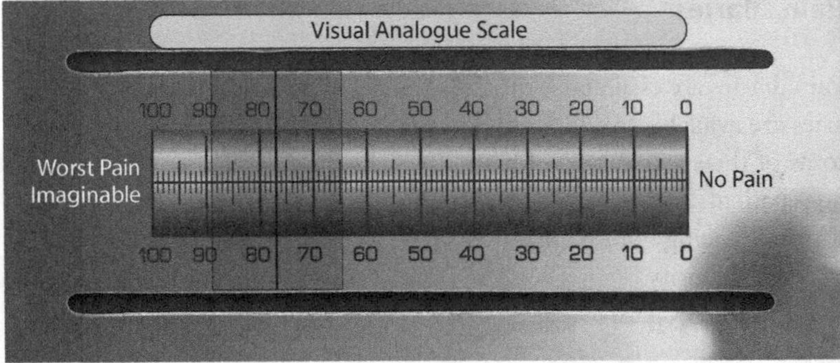

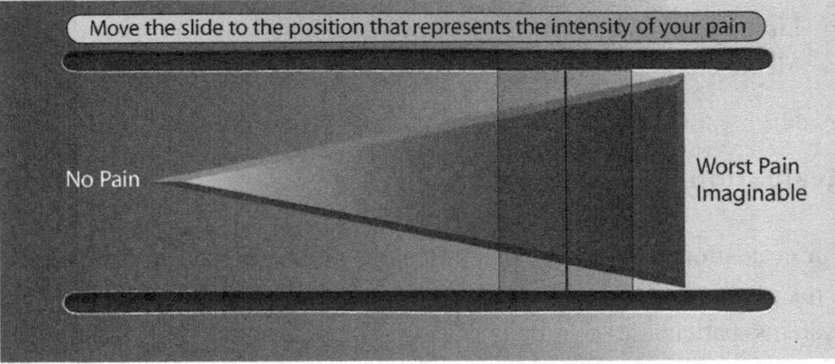

Fig. 1 Visual analogue scale

Numeric Rating Scale (NRS)

Patients relate their pain intensity to a rating number between pain free (0) and worst pain imaginable (10 or 100). This technique is more suitable for patients with a reduced level of cooperation.

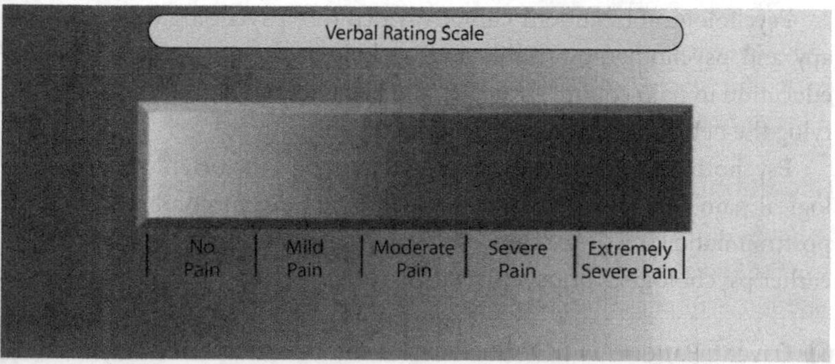

Fig. 2 Verbal rating scale

Verbal Rating Scale (VRS)

Patients are asked to relate their pain intensity to one out of five or more words (pain free to unbearable, Fig. 2). The main problem with this technique is that the adjectives trigger different associations in different patients. This technique therefore contains a systematic error and is less commonly used.

1.3 Psychological Pain Management

Knowledge about psychological and psychotherapeutic aspects of pain therapy are essential for the anesthetist working in this field. He should be able to explain the interplay of these factors to patients and thus prepare them for possible psychological treatment. Psychosocial diagnosis performed by a psychologist should evaluate the necessity of psychological therapy for the patient.

Psychological treatment can be divided into psychological pain therapy and psychotherapy (Table 1). Psychological pain therapy includes education in pain coping strategies and behavioral techniques and modifying the behavior that triggers and maintains pain.

Psychotherapy, as distinguished from symptom-orientated psychological pain therapy, is indicated for chronic pain in combination with posttraumatic stress reactions or chronic pain on the background of an earlier psychological or psychiatric disorder.

! Caveat: Patients with tendencies to somatization are often convinced that their pain has a purely organic origin, even if multiple examinations show no relevant organic defects. It is often impossible to convince these patients about the necessity of psychotherapeutic measures. In these cases it is often useful to try to convince them to learn how to improve their day-to-day level of function, including in relationships and about pain coping strategies as a first step. As a second and later step they should start psychotherapy.

Table 1 Psychological pain therapy versus psychotherapy for chronic pain

	Psychological pain therapy	Psychotherapy
Indication	Maladaptive pain and stress coping mechanisms	Psychological disorders as co-morbidity of chronic pain
	Psychosocial problems caused by chronic pain	Pain as symptom of a psychological disorder
		Psychosocial problems as main trigger for the pain disorder
Techniques	Pain coping strategies: – Psycho education – Relaxation (imagination techniques, progressive muscle relaxation (Jacobsen), biofeedback) – Cognitive strategies – Behavioral training	Behavioral therapy Psychoanalytic-oriented therapy Psychoanalytic-oriented therapy
	Stress coping strategies	Pain coping strategies for motivation to do psycho-therapy
Goals	Development of an adequate pain model Changes in pain perception Pain medication dose reduction Improvement of quality of life Adequate management of the pain disorder Modification of pain triggers	Treatment of the psychological disorder (causing the pain)
Setting	Single therapy/group therapy Inpatient or outpatient	Single therapy/group therapy Inpatient or outpatient

Bibliography

Institute for Clinical Systems Improvement (2007) Health care guideline: assessment and management of chronic pain, 2nd edn. ICSI, Bloomington (available at www.icsi.org)

Joint Commission on Accreditation of Healthcare Organizations (2000) Pain assessment and management: an organizational approach. Joint Commission Resources, Oakbrook Terrace

Kerns RD, Turk DC, Rudy TE (1985) The West Haven-Yale Multidimensional Pain Inventory (WHYMPI). Pain 23:345–356

Turk DC, Melzack R (2001) Handbook of pain assessment, 2nd edn. Guilford Press, New York

2 Headache

M. Schenk, H. Urnauer, S.A. Schug,
G. Jaehnichen, S.J. Harper

Classification

Headache can be classified into 14 groups according to the International Classification of Headache Disorders of the International Headache Society (IHS).

Epidemiology

- Migraine and tension-type headache constitute 92% of all headaches
- Lifetime incidence of headache is around 80%

Diagnostic Criteria

It is extremely important to exclude underlying pathology as a cause of headache. The criteria of the IHS classification provide a useful framework for diagnosis. The use of questionnaires can be helpful. The first assessment of head pain can be time-consuming, and might need to be performed repeatedly.

Headache diaries should be used for observation of disease progression. This is especially helpful for evaluation of therapy outcome, as well as for audit and quality control.

2.1 Migraine

Classification

IHS Codes 1.1–1.6

Diagnostic Criteria

Migraine without Aura

- At least 5 headache attacks, each lasting 4–72 h (untreated)
- Unilateral pain
- Pulsating pain quality
- Pain of medium to severe intensity
- Daily activities affected or impossible
- Intensely aggravated by physical activity
- Associated symptoms are nausea and/or vomiting, photophobia and phonophobia

Migraine with Aura

- See "Migraine without Aura" (above)
- In addition, neurological symptoms that develop over 5–20 min and last for < 1 h
- These symptoms correspond with brainstem or cerebral cortex processes

Typical Aura

- Homonymous visual disturbances
- Dysphasia
- Unilateral symptoms, e.g. impairment of sensibility or hemiplegia
- Duration < 1 h

Prolonged Aura

- Duration > 1 h and < 1 week

Familial Hemiplegic Migraine

- A first-degree family member has identical attacks

Basilar-Type Migraine

- Aura symptoms that can be linked to the brainstem or the occipital lobe

Status Migrainosus

- Duration under treatment longer than 72 h

Epidemiology

- Uniform worldwide prevalence, with a lifetime prevalence of 16% and a 1-year prevalence of 10%
- Male-female ratio of 1:2
- Average attack frequency of 3 days/month
- Increased prevalence with age until peak prevalence is reached during the fourth decade of life

Etiology

- Unknown
- Assumed dysfunction of neuronal mitochondria combined with increased neuronal excitability
- Underlying genetic mechanisms

Pathophysiology

The Vascular Theory

Trigeminal-mediated perivascular (neurogenic) inflammation leading to painful vascular and meningeal tissue. Wolffe suggested that early vasoconstriction of intra- and extracranial vessels gives rise to the aura preceding a migraine. The ensuing vasodilatation and increased blood flow are thought to cause headache via activation of the trigeminal sensory nerves that surround the meningeal blood vessels, causing pain. Activation of trigeminal nerves also causes the release of vasoactive neuropeptides that further contribute to dilation and worsen pain.

The Cortical Spreading Depression Theory

Cortical spreading depression (CSD) involves a brief wave of excitation followed by a prolonged period of neuronal depression that is associated with disturbances in nerve cell metabolism and regional reductions in blood flow. CSD passing forward over the cerebral cortex has been suggested as the cause of migraine aura.

The Neurovascular Hypothesis

The neurovascular hypothesis proposes that either migraine triggers or CSD can activate trigeminal nerve axons, which then release neuropeptides (such as substance P, neurokinin A and CGRP) from axon terminals near the meningeal and other blood vessels. These factors cause vasodilation and promote the extravasation of plasma proteins and fluid from nearby meningeal blood vessels, producing a perivascular inflammatory response. This response is termed sterile neurogenic perivascular inflammation.

The neuropeptides may also sensitize nerve endings, providing a mechanism for sustaining the headache. The activated trigeminal nerve also transmits pain impulses via the trigeminal nucleus caudalis to higher centers of the brain.

According to this theory, vasodilation is not the cause, but an accompanying phenomenon attributable to trigeminal nerve activation.

The Serotonergic Abnormalities Hypothesis

Both plasma and platelet levels of serotonin fluctuate during a migraine attack, which suggests that serotonin may be involved in the pathogenesis of migraine. When platelets are activated, they aggregate and release serotonin, thus increasing the plasma serotonin level. An increase in plasma serotonin level would be expected to cause vasoconstriction, whereas a decrease in serotonin would promote vasodilation.

Platelet serotonin levels may drop precipitously during the headache phase of migraine. Also, levels of serotonin and metabolites in urine rise during headaches, suggesting that there is a large release of serotonin during such attacks.

An initial surge in plasma serotonin levels may cause constriction of cerebral blood vessels and a reduction in cerebral blood flow. A subsequent depletion and drop in serotonin levels may then lead to a marked dilation of extracranial and intracranial arteries, precipitating migraine pain.

It has been suggested that the raphe nucleus, which is responsive to changes in serotonin levels, may serve as a "migraine generator."

The Integrated Hypothesis

This hypothesis attempts to consolidate the above theories and account for common observations about migraine headache such as trigger factors and response to treatment.

Differential Diagnosis

- Symptomatic (secondary) headache
- Cerebral ischemia
- Other primary headache types

Drug Therapy

Mild Migraine Attack

Nausea, Gastrointestinal Atonia

- Metoclopramide (1st line)
  Dose: 10–20 mg, 8 hourly PRN iv/im/po
- Domperidone (2nd line)
  Dose: 10 mg, 4 hourly PRN po (max 80 mg in 24 hours)

Analgesia

- Aspirin (1st line)
  Dose: 1000 mg, 4 hourly PRN po (max 4 g in 24 hours)
- Ibuprofen (2nd line)
  Dose: 400–800 mg, 6 hourly PRN po/pr (max 1600 mg in 24 hours)
- Paracetamol (2nd line)
  Dose: 1000 mg, 4 hourly PRN po/pr (max 4–6 g, according to national standards in 24 hours)

Severe Migraine Attack

Mild Nausea without Vomiting

- Sumatriptan
  Dose: 50–100 mg po/spray/iv at onset, repeated if symptoms recur (max 300 mg in 24 hours)
- Zolmitriptan
  Dose: 2.5 mg po repeated after 2 hours if symptoms persist (max 10 mg in 24 hours)

Severe Nausea with Vomiting

- Sumitriptan
  Dose: 6 mg s.c. 10–20 mg nasal, 25 mg rectal
- Zolmitriptan
  Dose: 2.5–5 mg s/l

Tab 2.1 Effectiveness of medications to abort acute migraine attacks. (From Australian and New Zealand College of Anaesthetists, Faculty of Pain Medicine. Acute pain management: scientific evidence. 2nd ed. Melbourne: Australian and New Zealand College of Anasthetists 2005.)

Agent	No. of studies	No. of total patients	Clinical success rate (%)	NNT: Clinical success# (95% CI)	Level of evidence
Chlorpromazine	*6*	*189*	*85*	*1.67 (1.53–1.85)*	*II*
Sumatriptan	*1*	*88*	*75*	*2 (1.72–2.5)*	*II*
Prochlorperazine	*3*	*70*	*76*	*2 (1.67–2.5)*	*II*
Metoclopramide	*4*	*121*	*59*	*2.9 (2.38–4)*	*II*
Ketorolac	*4*	*75*	*57*	*3.11 (2.27–4.76)*	*II*

Drug Therapy for Emergency Situations (Status Migrainosus)

- Metoclopramide
  Dose: 10–20 mg iv
- Alternative: Sumatriptan
  Dose: 6 mg sc or 1–2 mg Dihydroergotamine sc
- Parecoxib
  Dose: 40 mg iv/im once
- Dexamethasone
  Dose: 24 mg po/iv
- Frusemide
  Dose: 10 mg iv

Medical Prophylaxis

This is justified for severe migraine attacks with a high attack rate and severe impairment of daily living and performance at work. Mechanisms of action for medical prophylaxis are not yet known.

- Propanolol (1st line)
  Dose: 200 mg po/day
- Metoprolol (1st line)
  Dose: 200 mg po/day
- Flunarizine (ca-channel blocker used commonly in parts of Europe) (2nd line)
  Dose: 5–10 mg po/day

Interventional Pain Therapy

- Not indicated

Psychological Therapy and Prophylaxis

- Interval prophylaxis
  Stress management and relaxation training
  - Progressive muscle relaxation (Jacobsen), hypnosis
  - Cognitive behavioral therapy—efficacy well proven
- Treatment of the acute attack

Biofeedback: Vasoconstrictor training (efficacy well-proven, especially in connection with cognitive behavioral therapy), skin temperature training

Complementary Therapy

- Acupuncture

Physical Therapies

- Massage
- Peppermint oil in ethanol solution
- Physiotherapy
- Physical activity (aerobic exercises)

2.2 Tension-Type Headache (TTH)

Classification

IHS Codes 2.1–2.4

- Episodic TTH (IHS Codes 2.1 and 2.2):
  Headache on less than 15 days per month, or less than 180 days per year, with a duration from minutes to days.

- Chronic TTH (IHS Code 2.3):
  Headache on at least 15 days per month in at least 6 months per year, or on more than 180 days per year.

Diagnostic Criteria

- Pain of dull, tender, non pulsating quality
- Bilaterally localized pain in the neck/occipital region or frontal region
- Pain of low to medium intensity
- Tender pericranial muscles
- Marginal or absent vegetative symptoms
- No increase in pain intensity with physical activities

Epidemiolgy

- Most common type of headache
- Acute TTH prevalence: 40%–90%
- Chronic TTH prevalence: 3%
- Male-female ratio of 4:5

Etiology

- Tenderness in pericranial muscles, oromandibular dysfunction
- Anxiety or depression commonly co-exists (prevalence of 70%)
- Emotional conflict and psychosocial stress
- Medicine abuse

Pathophysiology

- Disorder of pericranial muscles and tendons with tenderness; initial muscular hypoxia and later microlesions
- Central chronification caused by chronic pain with activation of supraspinal pain perception structures

Differential Diagnosis

- Symptomatic (secondary) headache
- Other primary headache types

Drug Therapy

Episodic TTH

- Ibuprofen
  Dose: 400–800 mg, 6 hourly PRN po/pr (max 1600 mg in 24 hours)
- Paracetamol
  Dose: 500–1000 mg, 4–6 hourly PRN po/pr (max 4–6 g, according to national standards in 24 hours)
- Aspirin
  Dose: 500–1000 mg, 4 hourly PRN po (max 4 g in 24 hours)

! Advise pain medicine administration on not more than 10 days per month.

Chronic TTH

- Use no analgesics
- Amitriptyline (1st line)
  Dose: 10–25–50 mg po/day

- Doxepin (2nd line)
  Dose: 25–150 mg po/day (max 300 mg in 24 hours)

Interventional Pain Therapy

- Occipital and supraorbital nerve blocks

Psychological Therapy and Prophylaxis

- Progressive muscle relaxation and EMG-biofeedback
- Cognitive behavioral therapy

Complementary Therapy

- Acupuncture
- TENS

Physical Therapy

- Treatment of oromandibular dysfunction
- Hot and cold packs
- Massage
- Peppermint oil in ethanol solution
- Physiotherapy

! Non-pharmacological treatment options are of utmost importance for tension-type headaches.

2.3 Persistent Idiopathic Facial Pain

Classification

IHS Code 13.18.4—Diagnosis by exclusion.

Diagnostic Criteria

- Chronic pain, with possible additional attacks
- Pain of burning, throbbing and boring character
- Localization difficult, often unilateral, not consistent with known neurological pathways
- Often associated with anxiety and depression

Etiology

- Not known
- A diagnosis of exclusion
- Triggered by psychogenic factors

Epidemiology

- Highest prevalence after 30 years of age
- Male-female ratio of 2:8

Pathophysiology

- Not known
- Possible form of tension-type headache with facial localization

Differential Diagnosis

- Symptomatic (secondary) headache
- Other primary headache types
- Exclusion diagnosis

Drug Therapy

- Amitriptyline (1st line)
  Dose: 10–25–75 mg po/day
- Doxepin (2nd line)
  Dose: 10–75 mg po/day
- Carbamazepine
  Dose: 200–1200 mg po/day
- Tizanidine
  Dose: 3 × 2–8 mg po/day

Interventional Pain Therapy

- Stellate ganglion block

Psychological Therapy and Prophylaxis

- EMG-biofeedback
- Autosuggestive therapy
- Psychotherapy

Complementary Therapy

- Acupuncture
- TENS (transcutaneous electrical nerve stimulation)

Neurodestructive Procedures

- Contraindicated

! The face has very high density innervation. Facial pain has a high emotional component and therefore an increased risk of chronification. Invasive therapy may worsen the pain.

Psychogenic disorders such as depression, hypochondriasis, personality disorder, or abnormal illness behavior can often be found to coexist, but are commonly denied by patients. Psychotherapy is often helpful.

Important: Unnecessary dental and orofacial surgery procedures must be prevented.

2.4 Cluster Headache

Classification

IHS Code 3.1–3.4

- Episodic cluster headache (IHS Code 3.1.1):
  Cluster periods of between 1 week and 1 year, with pain-free intervals of 6 to 24 months.

- Chronic cluster headache (IHS Code 3.1.2):
  Cluster periods longer than 1 year without pain-free intervals of at least 14 days.

Diagnostic Criteria

- At least 5 attacks per month
- Up to 8 attacks per day on alternate days
- Duration of 15–180 min (untreated)
- Severe pain of boring and burning quality
- Severe to unbearable pain intensity
- Localization unilateral, periorbital, sometimes with occipital referral
- Accompanied by lacrimation, nasal drainage, pupillary changes and conjunctival injection
- Triggered by alcohol, vasodilators (nitroglycerine), or calcium antagonists

Epidemiology

- Prevalence around 1%
- Male-female ratio of 9:1
- Peak prevalence at 30 years of age

Etiology

- Not known

Pathophysiology

- Possible aseptic inflammation in the area of the cavernous sinus or superior ophthalmic vein, with following inflammatory alteration of bordering structures, such as the ophthalmic nerve

Differential Diagnosis

- Chronic paroxysmal hemicrania (Sjaastad syndrome)
- Symptomatic (secondary) headache
- Trigeminal neuralgia
- SUNCT syndrome (short-lasting unilateral neuralgia from headache attacks with conjunctival injection and tearing)

Drug Therapy

Drug Therapy during Attacks

- Sumatriptan
  Dose: 6 mg sc with auto injector; success rate: 74%

Additional Therapy during Attacks

- Oxygen
  Inhalation of 100% oxygen (6–8 l/min for 15 minutes)

Drug Therapy for Prophylaxis of Episodic Cluster Headache

- Verapamil (1st line)
  Dose: 240–360 mg, 12 hourly po or
- Ergotamine tartrate (1st line)
  Dose: 2–4 mg, 12 hourly po/pr

- Prednisolone (2nd line)
  Dose: 50 mg, 12 hourly po only short-term therapy
- Lithium (2nd line)
  Dose: 400 mg daily or 12 hourly po
- Methysergide malate (2nd line)
  Dose: 1–2 mg, 8–12 hourly po (2–3 week break required after 6 months continuous administration)

Drug Therapy for Prophylaxis of Chronic Cluster Headache

- Verapamil (1st line)
  Dose: 240–360 mg, 12 hourly po
- Lithium (1st line)
  Dose: 400 mg, daily or 12 hourly po
- Prednisolone (2nd line)
  Dose: 50 mg, 12 hourly po

Interventional Pain Therapy

- Blockade of the maxillary nerve and the pterygopalatine ganglion

Psychological Therapy

- Not primarily indicated

❗ Pharmacological treatment is of primary importance, as psychological factors are only of marginal relevance here.

2.5 Medication-Overuse Headache (MOH)

Classification

IHS Code 8.2.

Diagnostic Criteria

- Headache on at least 15 days per month
- Often daily, constant headache
- Pain of dull, tender, sometimes pulsating quality
- Accompanied by: nausea, vomiting, photophobia, phonophobia, tiredness and sleeping disorders
- Daily use of analgesics for more than 3 months, and pain relief within a month after cessation of analgesics
- After withdrawal of analgesics a severe withdrawal headache is common

Epidemiology

- No good data on prevalence available
- Male-female ratio of around 1:4

Etiology

- Analgesic-overuse headache:
  Monthly intake of at least 50 g aspirin or a similar analgesic (NSAIDS Paracetamol) or at least 100 tablets of a combination drug containing

barbiturates or other non-opioid analgesics or more than one opioid analgesic

- Ergotamine-overuse headache:
  Daily intake of 2 mg oral/1 mg rectal ergotamine tartrate. Combination drugs, especially containing caffeine, seem to have a very high potency

Pathophysiology

- Regular intake of high doses of analgesics in combination with psychotropic drugs (e. g. caffeine) leads to downregulation of pain receptor sensitivity
- Accompanied by changes in pain perception (hyperalgesia) caused by dysfunction of the antinociceptive system

Differential Diagnosis

- Symptomatic (secondary) headache
- Other primary headache types

Withdrawal Therapy

- Patients must be taught that analgesic drugs induce the headache
- Withdrawal therapy should preferably be performed in a specialized pain clinic over at least 14 days. Attempts of outpatient withdrawal therapy are often unsuccessful
- 40% of patients have a relapse within a year
- After successful withdrawal, the primary headache should be treated

Drug Therapy

- For reduction of vegetative withdrawal symptoms, antidepressive or neuroleptic drugs in low doses may be used
- Amitriptyline
  Dose: 25–75 mg po/day

Interventional Pain Therapy

- Not indicated

Psychological Therapy

- Prophylaxis through education, relaxation training and behavioral therapy

2.6 Trigeminal Neuralgia

Classification

IHS Code 13.1.

Diagnostic Criteria

- Paroxysmal pain attacks, of duration from seconds up to 2 minutes

- Superficial pain of stabbing, burning, shooting, electric shock-like quality
- Unilateral pain, localized in the trigeminal area (one or more branches of the trigeminal nerve)
- Pain attacks often caused by trigger factors such as cold, touch, stress
- No neurologic deficit
- Pain of severe intensity

Epidemiology

- Highest prevalence between 40 and 60 years of age
- Male-female ratio of 1:2

Etiology

- Compression and lesion of the trigeminal nerve caused by small tumors or blood vessels

Differential Diagnosis

- Symptomatic (secondary) headache
- Other primary headache types

Pathophysiology

- Remains poorly explained

- Caused by compression and subsequent demyelination of the trigeminal nerve at its entry into the pons. This is followed by increased afferent A- and C-fibre activity

Drug Therapy

- Carbamazepine (1st line)
  Dose: 200–400 mg daily in divided doses. Increase by 200 mg/day until pain relieved (maximum 1600 mg in 24 hours). Success rate over 80% in first-treatment patients
- Baclofen (2nd line)
  Dose: 5–25 mg, 8 hourly po. Success rate over 70% in first-treatment patients
- Phenytoin (2nd line)
  Dose: 100–300 mg daily in divided doses po. Success rate over 60% in first-treatment
- Clonazepam (3rd line)
  Dose: 0.5–2 mg, 6–12 hourly po (max 8 mg in 24 hours)
- Gabapentin
  Dose: 300–900 mg, 8 hourly (titrated to effect as tolerated)
- Lamotrigine
  Dose: 50 mg daily for 2 weeks, then increase to 100 mg daily for two weeks and thereafter by 100 mg every two weeks (max 400 mg daily in divided doses)
- Combination therapy including some or all of the above
  Dose: see above

Interventional Pain Therapy

- Local anesthetic blockade of peripheral branches of the trigeminal nerve, followed perhaps by neurolysis:
  - V 1: Supraorbital nerve, supratrochlear nerve
  - V 2: Maxillary nerve (including pterygopalatine ganglion), infraorbital nerve
  - V 3: Mandibular nerve (including otical ganglion), mental nerve

Psychological Therapy and Prophylaxis

- Psychotherapy for treatment of the often coexisting depression
- Support and education

Invasive Therapy

- Surgical procedures: microvascular decompression, gamma knife radiosurgery

Trigeminal neuralgia remains incurable; therapy with analgesics is always a long-term prospect. After initially successful analgesic therapy, in many cases the efficacy of the pain medicine decreases.

Bibliography

Lipton RB, Bigal ME, Steiner TJ, Silberstein SD, Olesen J (2004) Classification of primary headaches. Neurology 63:427–435

Institute for Clinical Systems Improvement (2007) Health care guideline: diagnosis and treatment of headache. ICSI, Bloomington (available at www.icsi.org)

Olesen J, Goadsby PJ, Ramadan NM, Tfelt-Hansen P, Welch KMA (2006) The headaches, 3rd edn. Lippincott Williams & Wilkins, Philadelphia

Lance JW, Goadsby PJ (2005) Mechanism and management of headache, 7th edn. Elsevier, Butterworth, Heinemann, Philadelphia

Marcus DA (2007) Headache and chronic pain syndromes: the case-based guide to targeted assessment and treatment. Humana Press, Totowa

Websites

www.i-h-s.org: website of the International Headache Society, providing detailed guidelines on the classification of headache based on the best currently available evidence.

www.headaches.org: website of the US-based National Headache Foundation, which provides up-to-date information on diagnosis, treatment and research into headaches, as well as downloadable assessment tools.

3 Pain of Musculoskeletal Origin

M. Schenk, H. Urnauer, S.A. Schug, G. Jaehnichen, S.J. Harper

3.1 Back Pain

Classification (ICD 10, SGB-V, Version 2.0)

M 54.1 Radiculopathy
M 54.2 Cervical Neuralgia
M 54.3 Ischialgia
M 54.4 Lumbar Ischialgia
M 54.5 Backache
M 54.6 Pain of the Thoracic Spine
M 54.8 Other Back Pain
M 54.9 Chronic Back Pain

Epidemiology

Prevalence statistics about back pain:

- 20.9% of population self-reported having back pain or disc disorders in Australia in 2001 (ABS 2001 National Health Survey, Australia's Health 2004, AIHW)
- 20.7% of female population self-reported having back pain or disc disorders in Australia in 2001 (ABS 2001 National Health Survey, Australia's Health 2004, AIHW)
- 21.0% of male population self-reported having back pain or disc disorders in Australia in 2001 (ABS 2001 National Health Survey, Australia's Health 2004, AIHW)
- 3,937,000 people self-reported having back pain or disc disorders in Australia in 2001 (ABS 2001 National Health Survey, Australia's Health 2004, AIHW)
- 1,944,000 men self-reported having back pain or disc disorders in Australia in 2001 (ABS 2001 National Health Survey, Australia's Health 2004, AIHW)

- 1,993,000 women self-reported having back pain or disc disorders in Australia in 2001 (ABS 2001 National Health Survey, Australia's Health 2004, AIHW)

Incidence and Prevalence

In the United States, back pain is reported to occur at least once in 85% of adults below the age of 50. Nearly all of them will have at least one recurrence. It is the second most common illness-related reason given for a missed workday, and the most common cause of disability. Work-related back injury is the number one occupational hazard.

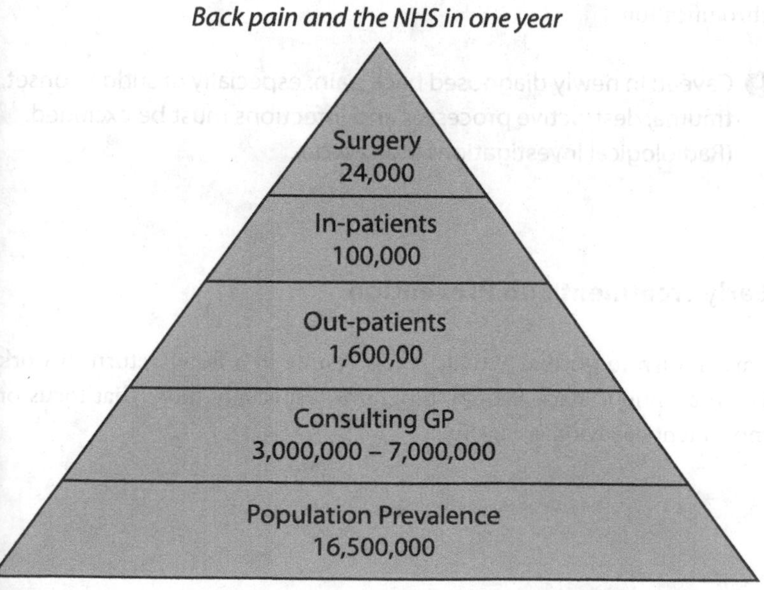

Fig. 3 The Back-Pain Pyramid (numbers from National Health Service UK)

Biopsychosocial model vs. Anatomical model

Because the biopsychosocial model explains the discrepancy between objective disability and subjective impairment it should be favored. In around 90% of patients with back pain, no distinct anatomical diagnosis can be made and the final diagnosis will be non-specific back pain (or similar term). Examination of patients with radiculopathy in an acute stage versus 6 months after onset of pain revealed risk factors for chronification of pain (mechanical/psychological stress, fear-avoidance behavior, negative emotions).

Further psychosocial factors with a high predictive value are psychiatric disorders (depression, anxiety disorders, somatic fixation) and dissatisfaction in the workplace. A multidisciplinary approach, including psychotherapeutic measures, is helpful in cases that are high risk for chronification.

! Caveat: In newly diagnosed back pain, especially of sudden onset, trauma, destructive processes and infections must be excluded. (Radiological investigations indicated.)

Early Treatment and Prevention

Early return to normal activity levels results in a faster return to work For prevention, 'Back School' programs, especially those that focus on movement behavior, are useful.

Multimodal Therapy of Chronic Back Pain

Includes:

- Exercise
- Behavioral therapy
- Occupational therapy (Therapy aimed at the development, recovery and/or maintenance of individual daily routines. It involves targeted use of selected activities to analyze and treat consequences of disease and/or disability.)

Meta-analyses show that a multimodal approach, utilizing the skills of a variety of professionals, is preferable. Group training in pain coping and behavioral strategies, as well as exercise classes combined with relaxation and education sessions, have been shown to be effective.

3.2 Radicular Root Irritation Syndrome

Diagnostic Criteria

- Compression/Irritation of the nerve root caused by a prolapsed intervertebral disc
- Mostly sudden, well-defined onset
- Well-defined pain location, often affecting one or more dermatomes with pain shooting into the legs
- Severe pain of burning, stabbing or electric shock-like quality, together with diminished reflexes and hyperalgesia. Pain triggered by pressing, coughing or certain movements
- Investigations:
  Electromyography is the investigation of choice. It is sensitive from two weeks after the lesion, and allows old and new root lesions to be distinguished. However, the therapeutic implications are limited.

- Imaging:
  Often low correlation between patients' pain and result of imaging studies

Etiology

- Prolapsed intervertebral disc

Pathophysiology

- Irritation by local inflammatory response to extruded disc material
- Nerve root compression is of secondary importance
- Secondary pain caused by muscle spasms

Differential Diagnosis

- Pseudoradicular root irritation syndrome
- Degenerative disease of the sacroiliac joints
- Degenerative disease of the facet joints
- Hypermobility
- Infective or destructive processes
- Central or peripheral spinal stenosis
- Neurological disorders
- Peripheral nerve compression syndromes

Drug Therapy

- Diclofenac

Dose: 50–100 mg, 8 to 12 hourly po/pr (max 150 mg in 24 h) max 3 weeks
- Parecoxib
  Dose: 40 mg daily, 12 hourly iv
- Prednisolone
  Dose: 30 mg daily po for 5 days NB: In severe cases, specific treatment of neuopathic pain with anticonvulsans or antidepressants may be indicated!

Interventional Pain Therapy

- Lumbar epidural steroid injections
  Dose: Ropivacaine 0.2% 10 ml and Triamcinolone 80 mg
- Lumbar sympathetic blocks
- Paravertebral blocks
- Nerve root sleeve injections

Complementary Therapy

- Acupuncture
- Low frequency TENS (2–10 Hz)

Physical Therapy

- Early physiotherapy
- Back School
- Occupational therapy
- Massage
- Traction and bed rest are not indicated

Psychological Therapy and Prophylaxis

Prevention of chronification:

- Behavioral training especially designed for the workplace
- Relaxation training

❗ The role of manipulation and chiropractic treatment is important. Curative therapy may be possible.

3.3 Pseudoradicular Root Irritation Syndrome

Diagnostic Criteria

- Chronic onset
- Pain quality diffuse, difficult to localize, dull
- Often located on both sides of the body
- Triggered by pain/trigger points?

Epidemiology

- See above

Etiology

- Arthropathy of the sacroiliac joints (sacroiliac joint disease/irritation of nerve roots at the sacroiliac joints)
- Facet joint disease in the lower lumbar spine affecting the function of joints and muscles
- Hypermobility

- Leg length inequality
- Peripheral nerve compression syndromes
- Correlation with depression and anxiety disorders
- Neuromuscular imbalance

Pathophysiology

- Disorder of the functional spinal unit, secondary muscular spasm and neurological deficits

Differential Diagnosis

- Radicular root irritation syndrome
- Infective or destructive processes

Drug Therapy

- Amitriptyline (1st line)
  Dose: 25–75 mg nocte
- Doxepin (2nd line)
  Dose: 10–75 mg po/day
- In severe pain short term use of Morphine, Fentanyl, Tramadol, Buprenorphine, Oxycodone or Hydromorphone (slow release if possible)
  Dose: Titrate to effect

Interventional Pain Therapy

(If effective and no psychosocial contraindications)

- Paravertebral nerve block
- Epidural anesthesia

Complementary Therapy

- Acupuncture
- Low frequency TENS (2–10 Hz)

Physical Therapy

- Manipulation
- Physiotherapy
- Back School
- Ergotherapy
- Massage

Psychological Therapy and Prophylaxis

- Behavioral training
- Relaxation training
- Progressive muscle relaxation (Jacobsen)
- Hypnosis
- Biofeedback
- Physical paced aerobic activation

! The role of manipulation and chiropractic treatment is important. Curative therapy may be possible.

3.4 Fibromyalgia

Classification (ICD 10, SGB-V, Version 2.0)

M 79.0 Rheumatism, Fibromyalgia, Fibromyalgia syndrome

Diagnostic Criteria

- Widespread pain in multiple regions
- More than 3 months duration
- Tenderness on bilateral palpation of at least 11 out of 18 classic tender points (Wolfe 1990)
- Exclusion of other medical conditions
- Low serotonin and tryptophane blood levels and high substance P CSF levels

Epidemiology

- 1% of population
- Women more often affected than men

Etiology

- Not known
- Patients with fibromyalgia have an increased incidence of psychological disorders compared to chronic arthritis patients or healthy controls
- Increased prevalence of depression, but incidence of coexistent psychosis similar to other chronic pain syndromes

Pathophysiology

- Not known, central nervous system sensitization most likely explanation
- Increased levels of substance P, hormone regulation dysfunction

Drug Therapy

- Amitriptyline
  Dose: 25–50 mg po/day
- Tramadol slow release
  Dose: 3 × 50–200 mg po/day
- Gabapentin
  Dose: 3 × 100–900 mg po/day
- Pregabalin
  Dose: 2 × 75–300 mg po/day

Interventional Pain Therapy

- Not indicated

Psychological Therapy and Prophylaxis

- Psychotherapy, in particular treatment of any coexisting depression
- Pain coping skills training
- Cognitive-behavioral pain management (CBT)
- Paced physical aerobic activation

! A multimodal, multidisciplinary approach is important. Psychotherapy may be extremely helpful. Drug therapy often leads to a disappointingly small reduction in pain, but may permit participation in physical activity.

3.5 Osteoporosis

Classification (ICD 10, SGB-V, Version 2.0)

M 81 Osteoporosis without pathological fracture

Diagnostic Criteria

- Systemic disease of the skeleton with reduction in bone mass and increased fracture risk
- Bone pain is the leading clinical feature
- Often associated with neck, femur, arm and spine fractures
- Can be divided into postmenopausal type I and senile type II
- Diagnosis made with imaging techniques (reduction of bone mass of >30%) and measurement of bone density

Epidemiology

- Primary osteoporosis is the cause in 95% of cases, 80% in postmenopausal women

Etiology

- Primary osteoporosis:
  - Increasing age

- Female gender
- Inactivity
- Low levels of calcium and vitamin D, odd diets
- Smoking

Differential Diagnosis

- Malignant processes
- Primary hyperparathyroidism
- Osteomalacia

Drug Therapy

- Analgesic drugs titrated to effect using the analgesic ladder, i.e. simple analgesics, NSAIDS and weak opioids, then strong opioids if required
- Calcium
  Dose: 1000–1500 mg po/day
- Alendronate
  Dose: 10 mg po/day or 70 mg po/week
- Calcitonin
  Dose: 200 I.E. as nasal spray/iv/sc/day

Interventional Pain Therapy

- Vertebroplasty

Psychological Therapy and Prophylaxis

- Relaxation training
- Behavior modification
- Stress management

Bibliography

Abeles AM, Pillinger MH, Solitar BM, Abeles M (2007) Narrative review: the pathophysiology of fibromyalgia. Ann Intern Med 146:726–734

Carville SF, Arendt-Nielsen S, Bliddal H, Blotman F, Branco JC, Buskilla D, Da Silva JA, Danneskiold-Samsoe B, Dincer F, Henriksson C, Henriksson K, Kosek K, Longley K, McCarthy GM, Perrot S, Puszczewicz MJ, Sarzi-Puttini P, Silman A, Spath M, Choy EH (2007) EULAR evidence based recommendations for the management of fibromyalgia syndrome. Ann Rheum Dis doi:10.1136/ard.2007.071522

Freedman MK, Morrison WB, Harwood MI, (2007) Minimally invasive musculoskeletal pain medicine. Informa Healthcare, New York

Institute for Clinical Systems Improvement (2006) Health care guideline: diagnosis and treatment of osteoporosis, 5th edn. ICSI, Bloomington (available at www.icsi.org)

Institute for Clinical Systems Improvement (2006) Health care guideline: adult low back pain, 12th edn. ICSI, Bloomington (available at www.icsi.org)

Jenis LG (2005) American Academy of Orthopaedic Surgeons: Back pain, 1st edn. American Academy of Orthopaedic Surgeons, Rosemont

Levine JP (2006) Pharmacologic and nonpharmacologic management of osteoporosis. Clin Cornerstone 8:40–53

Marcus R (2007) Osteoporosis, 3rd edn. Academic Press, San Diego

Singer A (2006) Osteoporosis diagnosis and screening. Clin Cornerstone 8:9–18

Wallace DJ, Clauw DJ (2005) Fibromyalgia and other central pain syndromes. Lippincott Williams & Wilkins, Philadelphia

Wolfe F, Smythe HA, Yunus MB, Bennett RM, Bombardier C, Goldenberg DL, Tugwell P, Campbell SM, Abeles M, Clark P, et al. (1990) The American College of

Rheumatology 1990 Criteria for the Classification of Fibromyalgia. Report of the Multicenter Criteria Committee. Arthritis Rheum 33:160–172

Websites

www.g-i-n.net: International guideline library with links to many national guidelines on low back pain in the health topics collection.

4 Neuropathic Pain

*M. Schenk, H. Urnauer, S.A. Schug,
G. Jaehnichen, S.J. Harper*

Diagnostic Criteria

Pain of burning, lancinating, cutting, shooting, electric shock-like quality. Often superficially located and associated with allodynia, hyperaesthesia and trophic disorders.

Etiology

- Destruction of peripheral nerves, spinal cord or cerebrum
- Deafferentation pain with or without amputation. Amputation, neurolysis or a plexus lesion leads to increased activity of parts of the nociceptive system, i.e., central sensitization

Drug Therapy

Corticosteroids for nerve compression, carbamazepine, antidepressant drugs, gabapentin, clonazepam, opioids.

Psychological Therapy and Prophylaxis

- Hypnotic pain therapy
- Relaxation training
- Stress management
- All aimed at changing the patient's perception of the pain and its impact.

4.1 Complex Regional Pain Syndrome (CRPS)

Classification (ICD 10, SGB-V, Version 2.0)

M 89.0 Neurodystrophia (algodystrophy), shoulder-hand syndrome, Sudeck's dystrophy, reflex sympathetic dystrophy.

CRPS Type 1

Previously known as reflex sympathetic dystrophy (RSD).

CRPS Type 2

Previously known as causalgia. Identical to CRPS type 1, except that it is accompanied by a nerve lesion and neurological deficit.

Diagnostic Criteria

- Sensory disturbances (hypoaesthesia)
- Spontaneous burning pain, allodynia, hyperalgesia
- Motor dysfunction:
  - Muscle atrophia with reduction of strength and loss of motor function, including dystonia and tremor
- Sympathetic nervous system dysfunction:
  - Generalized swelling (oedema), trophic disorders, temperature changes, bleeding disorders
- Gravity dependent pain—related to increase in hydrostatic pressure
- Commonly localized to the distal extremities

- Pain relief may occur after ischemia testing or sympathetic nerve blocks
- Diagnosis is clinical; laboratory and radiological examinations are unhelpful
- Pseudo neglect phenomenon

Epidemiology

- Average age: 40 years
- Male-female ratio of 1:2

Etiology

- Trauma or surgical insult that may be relatively minor
- High level of anxiety, emotional lability, depression or exhaustion at the time of trauma

Pathophysiology

- Maintenance of pain via the sympathetic nervous system
- Common mechanism of chronification with spontaneous activity and peripheral (nociceptors) and central sensitization
- Neurogenic inflammation (antidromic)

Differential Diagnosis

- Delayed wound healing
- Atrophia due to inactivity
- In acute development, osteomyelitis/cellulitis

Drug Therapy

- Non-opioid analgesics, including NSAIDS
- Amitriptyline
  Dose: 10–25–75 mg po daily over 2 weeks
- Mirtazapine
  Dose: 30 mg po/day
- Prednisolone
  Dose: 40–80 mg po/day over 2 weeks
- Calcitonin
  Dose: 100–200 I.E. iv or nasal spray/day over 6 weeks
- Gabapentin
  Dose: 300–1800–3600 mg po/day
- Pregabalin
  Dose: 150–600 mg po/day
- Ketamine
  Continuous infusion started at 0.1 mg/kg/hr, to be titrated upwards to effect/adverse effects
- Slow release opioids (tramadol, morphine, methadone or oxycodone) according to the WHO Guidelines
  Dose: Titration

Interventional Pain Therapy

- Sympathetic nerve blocks
- Blocks of the inferior ganglion of the cervical sympathetic chain
- Plexus blocks, e. g. brachial, lumbar
- Lumbar epidural analgesia with clonidine
- Intravenous regional anesthesia with guanethidine
- Dorsal column stimulation (DCS)

Physical Therapy

- Physiotherapy
- Lymph drainage
- Ergotherapy

Psychological Therapy and Prophylaxis

- Sensory desensitization and discrimination training may help with neglect-like disorders; mirror box use and limb laterality recognition programs are part of such training
- Gentle exercise programmes, e.g. Tai Chi
- For acute symptoms:
  Rest, no unnecessary movements, but desensitization and discrimination training below pain threshold
- After resolution of acute symptoms:
  Stress management, prevention of overactivity, paced return to activity, emotional support

Complimentary Therapy

- Acupuncture
- TENS

! Often underdiagnosed or diagnosed at a late stage, can lead to a complete loss of function. End stage CRPS may require amputation of the affected limb, but this will not resolve pain. A multidisciplinary approach with coordination of pain therapy, physiotherapy and psychotherapy is advised.

4.2 Phantom Pain

Classification (ICD 10, SGB-V, Version 2.0)

G 54.6 Phantom Pain
G 54.7 Phantom Limb without Pain

Diagnostic Criteria

- Often constant pain
- Pain of burning, cramping, electric shock-like pain, stinging, shooting quality
- Very high pain intensity
- Phantom pain is a painful sensation in a body part that does not exist, e. g. has been amputated. (c.f. phantom sensation, which is non-painful)

Epidemiology

- 50%–85% after lower limb amputation

Etiology

- Amputation of parts of the body (e. g. limbs, breast, rectum, tongue)

Pathophysiology

- Deafferentation hypothesis:
  There is a lack of large fiber inhibition of excitatory neurons of central nociceptic systems in the spinal cord, thalamus and cortex caused by decreasing afferent input into the CNS due to deafferentiation
- Pain intensity also depends on cortical representation of amputated limb and on increase of the receptive fields adjoining the amputation site

Differential Diagnosis

- Stump pain

Drug Therapy

- Amitriptyline
  Dose: 10–25–150 mg po/day
- Gabapentin
  Dose: 300–3600 mg po/day
- Pregabalin
  Dose: 150–600 mg po/day
- Calcitonin
  Dose: 200 I.E. iv or nasal spray/day over 3–5 days
- Mexiletine
  Dose: 1 × 400 mg po/day initially, then 3 × 200 mg po/day
- Amantadine
  Dose: 200 mg iv over 3 hours, maybe continue with oral applications
- Ketamine

Dose: Continuous infusion started at 0.1 mg/kg/hr, to be titrated upwards to effect/adverse effects

- Opioids (tramadol, morphine, methadone or oxycodone) according to the WHO Guidelines
  Dose: Titration

Interventional Pain Therapy

- Perioperative continuous epidural anesthesia/analgesia has preventative effect for phantom pain
- Sympathetic nerve blocks:
  - Block of the inferior ganglion of the cervical sympathetic chain
  - Block of the lumbar sympathetic chain for the lower limbs
  - Epidural analgesia

Psychological Therapy

- Stress management and relaxation training
- Progressive muscle relaxation (Jacobsen technique)
- Hypnosis

Complementary Therapy

- Acupuncture
- Neural therapy
- TENS

! Therapy of chronic phantom pain is extraordinarily difficult. Meticulous attention to perioperative pain therapy is essential to reduce the incidence. The aim should be for a pain-free patient pre-amputation. Early use of calcitonin is the most effective treatment, should phantom pain develop.

4.3 Postherpetic Neuralgia

Classification (ICD 10, SGB-V, Version 2.0)

B. 02 Zoster (Herpes zoster)

Diagnostic Criteria

- Constant pain
- Pain of burning, boring or shooting quality
- Allodynia
- Pain of severe intensity
- Ocular complications may occur with damage to the facial nerve

Epidemiology

- Incidence in the elderly around 125 per 100,000/year
- Incidence increases with age and immunosuppression
- Male-female ratio of 1:1

Pathophysiology

- Follows infection with the varicella zoster virus. There is reactivation of latent virus by increased replication in nerve cells, especially those of the dorsal root ganglion (DRG) and cranial nerve nuclei. Viral necrotizing inflammation of myelinated nerve fibers with partial destruction leads to neuropathic pain and sometimes associated neurological deficits.

Differential Diagnosis

- Trigeminal neuralgia
- Intercostal neuralgia
- Atypical facial pain

Drug Therapy

Drug Therapy of Acute Zoster Pain

- Aciclovir
  Dose: 800 mg 5 times daily po or 5–10 mg/kg iv, 8 hourly for 7–10 days
- Famciclovir
  Dose: 250 mg po/day for 7 days

Early antiviral therapy reduces the risk of pain chronification.

- Amantadine
  Dose: 200–400 mg iv/day until pain intensity is decreasing
- Opioids, e.g. Oxycodone according to the WHO Guidelines
- Amitriptyline
  Dose: 10–25–50 mg po/day

! Early use of amitriptyline for 3 months reduces the risk of pain chronification.

Drug Therapy of Post Herpetic Neuralgia

- Lidocaine plaster 5%
  Apply topically over area of pain and allodynia for 12 to 24 hrs
- Amitriptyline
  Dose: 10–25–75 mg po/day
- Gabapentin
  Dose: 300–3600 mg po/day
- Pregabalin
  Dose: 150–600 mg po/day
- Opioids
  Dose and opioid type according to the WHO Guidelines
- Amantadine
  Dose: 100–200 mg po 12 hourly
- Capasaicin creme
  Dose: 2–4 times/day for 4–6 weeks
- EMLA creme
  Dose: 2–4 times/day for 4–6 weeks

Interventional Pain Therapy

Interventional Pain Therapy of Acute Zoster Pain

- Sympathetic nerve blocks
- Upper limbs:
  - Blocks of the superior ganglion of the cervical sympathetic chain
  - Blocks of the inferior ganglion of the cervical sympathetic chain
- Lower limbs:
  - Epidural catheters or lumbar sympathetic blocks

Interventional Pain Therapy of Post Herpetic Neuralgia

As for management of acute Zoster pain:

- Upper limbs: blockade of the inferior ganglion of the cervical sympathetic chain
- Lower limbs: Epidural analgesia with steroids or lumbar sympathetic blockade

Psychological Therapy and Prophylaxis

- Stress control and relaxation training
- Imagination techniques

Complimentary Therapy

- Acupuncture
- Neural therapy
- TENS

❗ Like other neuropathic pain syndromes, post herpetic neuralgia is difficult to treat after chronification. Antiviral therapy should be started early during the viral replication phase. Developing post herpetic pain must be treated quickly and aggressively. A series of sympathetic blocks seem to be especially effective.

Bibliography

Attal N, Cruccu G, Haanpaa M, Hansson P, Jensen TS, Nurmikko T, et al. (2006) EFNS guidelines on pharmacological treatment of neuropathic pain. Eur J Neurol. 13(11):1153–69.

Berthelot JM (2006) Current management of reflex sympathetic dystrophy syndrome (complex regional pain syndrome type I). Joint Bone Spine 73:495–499

Bowsher D. (1997) The effects of pre-emptive treatment of postherpetic neuralgia with amitriptyline: a randomized, double-blind, placebo-controlled trial. J Pain Symptom Manage 13(6):327–31.

Cunningham AL, Dworkin RH (2000) The management of post-herpetic neuralgia. BMJ 321:778–779

Finnerup NB, Otto M, McQuay HJ, Jensen TS, Sindrup SH (2005) Algorithm for neuropathic pain treatment: an evidence based proposal. Pain. ;118(3):289–305.

Flor H (2002) Phantom-limb pain: characteristics, causes and treatment. Lancet Neurol 1:182–189

Gilron I, Watson CP, Cahill CM, Moulin DE (2006) Neuropathic pain: a practical guide for the clinician. MAJ 175:265–275

Hansson P (2001) Neuropathic pain: pathophysiology and treatment. IASP Press, Seattle

Janig W, Baron R. (2003) Complex regional pain syndrome: mystery explained? Lancet Neurol. 2(11):687-97.

Jackson KC 2nd (2006) Pharmacotherapy for neuropathic pain. Pain Pract 6:27–33

Mailis A, Furlan A (2003) Sympathectomy for neuropathic pain. Cochrane Database Syst Rev CD002918

Manchikanti L, Singh V (2004) Managing phantom pain. Pain Physician 7:365–375

Rowbotham MC (2006) Pharmacologic management of complex regional pain syndrome. Clin J Pain 22:425–429

Visser EJ. (2005) A review of calcitonin and its use in the treatment of acute pain. Acute Pain. 7(4):185-9.

Websites

www.neupsig.org: Website of the special interest group on neuropathic pain of the International Association for the Study of Pain (IASP).

5 Cancer Pain

M. Schenk, H. Urnauer, S.A. Schug, G. Jaehnichen, S.J. Harper

Introduction and General Principles

Potentially curative therapy (surgery, chemotherapy, radiotherapy) is always the first line of treatment for cancer patients.

Cancer pain therapy is symptomatic therapy with the goal of effective reduction of pain (pain at rest VAS <3, pain at movement VAS <6) and preservation of a good quality of life (minimizing side effects of the pain therapy).

Cancer pain can be influenced negatively by psychological disorders and dysfunctional behavior. If cancer pain is not treated sufficiently, impairment of various aspects of quality of life affecting the progress of the disease and functional status of the patient are likely to occur.

Quality of life can also be reduced by inappropriate invasive pain therapy or inappropriate pharmacological therapy causing disabling side-effects.

Epidemiology

Incidence

Around 50% of all cancer patients have cancer pain; in the terminal stages it is more than 70%.

Intensity

50% of patients have medium to severe pain.
30% of patients describe the pain as unbearable at some times.
Up to 80% of patients with cancer pain receive inadequate pain therapy.

Classification by Etiology

Pain that occurs during cancer is divided into groups as follows:

Directly Tumor-Related—60%–90%

Caused by:

- Infiltration or compression of nerve tissue
- Soft tissue infiltration
- Infiltration of hollow viscera
- Invasion of bone or bony metastasis

Complications of Cancer Treatment—10%–25%

Caused by:

- Drugs
- Radiotherapy
- Post surgical syndrome

Cancer Associated—5%–20%

Caused by:

- Paraneoplastic syndrome
- Postural disturbance

Unrelated to Cancer—3%–10%

Classification of Type of Pain

Nociceptor Pain—Somatic

- Structures involved:
  Skin, muscles, bones, soft tissues
- Quality of pain:
  Easy to localize, stabbing, boring, movement-dependent

Nociceptor Pain—Visceral

- Structures involved:
  Parenchymatous organs, hollow viscera, peritoneum
- Quality of pain:
  Difficult to localize, dull, oppressive, colicky

Neuropathic Pain

- Structures involved:
  Nociceptic system (peripheral nerves, spinal cord, cerebrum)
- Quality of pain:
  Shooting, lancinating, electric shock-like, burning

Therapy—General Principles

Requirements

- Detailed evaluation of the patient's general history and pain history
- Pain therapy according to the guidelines for cancer pain of the WHO (see Fig. 4.)

WHO Step III

C – Opioid for moderate to severe pain
Morphine
Methadone
Oxycodone
Hydromorphone
Buprenorphine
Dextromoramide
± nonopioid
± adjuvants

WHO Step II ***If pain persists or increases***

B – Opioid for mild to moderate pain
Tramadol
Codeine
Dihydrocodeine
Dextropropoxyphene
± nonopioid
± adjuvants

WHO Step I ***If pain persists or increases***

A – Nonopioid
Acetaminophen
Dipyrone
NSAIDs
± adjuvants

Chemotherapy/Radiotherapy --
Physical/Psychological/Behavioral Therapy --------------------------
Empathy/Care --

Fig. 4 WHO Guidelines

Analgesics—Choice

- The choice of analgesics depends on the character, cause and severity of pain
- Opioids of WHO level II and III should not be combined

Analgesics—Administration

- Analgesics should be given orally if possible
- Transdermal analgesics should generally be administered after enteral or parenteral dose titration
- The formulation/route of administration that is most convenient for the patient should be chosen

Analgesics—Basic Medication

- Analgesics should be given in a slow release form according to a strict time regime
- Adjustment of the pain therapy should be done prospectively and not reactively, if possible

Analgesics—Supplemental Medication

- Pain therapy should always include immediate release medication for treatment of breakthrough pain

❶ Mistake: Supplemental medication only.

Analgesics—Therapy of Side Effects

- Side effects should be treated prophylactically where possible e.g., opioid administration should always be combined with laxative
- Any side effects should be carefully documented

Drug Therapy—Most Common Errors

Opioids

- Irrational fear of addiction and tolerance
- "Sparing" of opioids
- Patient refusal of opioids
- "Withdrawal treatment" of pain that requires opioids
- Irrational opioid combinations (agonists + partial antagonists)

Others

- Mixed analgesics
- Missing co-medication

WHO Guidelines for Treatment of Cancer Pain

The WHO Guidelines are not a rigid scheme for pain therapy, but a structure for single elements of pain therapy. Similar therapy measures are put into the different levels. The levels do not have to be used in any particular order, and they can generally be combined or supplemented (level II and III should not be combined). Patients with severe cancer pain might be treated with level III analgesics from the outset, without adding analgesics from level I. For all patients, an individual strategy for pain therapy should be developed.

Therapy with Non-opioid Analgesics (WHO Step I)

1. Cox-II inhibitors
- Indication: Nociceptive pain, especially of a somatic type
- Dose:

  Parecoxib: 2×40 mg iv/day

  Celecoxib: 2×100–200 mg po/day

2. Paracetamol
- Indication: Nociceptive pain
- Dose: 8 × 500–1000 mg po/day or 4 × 1 g iv (Perfalgan) in 24 hours

3. NSAIDS
- Indication: Nociceptive pain, especially of a somatic type with an inflammatory component
- Dose:

Ibuprofen:	3 × 400–800 mg po/day
Diclofenac:	3 × 50 mg po or rectal/day
Naproxen:	2 × 250–500 mg po/day

Therapy with Opiods (WHO Steps II and III)

1. Tilidine + Naloxone slow-release
- Indication: Basic analgesia (WHO level II)
- Route: po
- Dose: Demand-orientated, 150–600 mg/day; 2–3 doses/day

2. Tramadol slow-release
- Indication: Basic analgesia, WHO level II
- Route: po
- Dose: Demand-orientated, 150–600 mg/day; 2–3 doses/day

3. Morphine sulphate slow release
- Indication: Basic analgesia (gold standard)
- Route: po
- Dose: Demand-orientated, 2–3 doses/day

4. Morphine sulphate–granulate slow release
- Indication: Basic analgesia, WHO level III; if problems swallowing tablets
- Route: po
- Dose: Demand-orientated, 2–3 doses/day

5. Hydromorphone slow release
- Indication: Basic analgesia, WHO level III
- Route: po or via PEG with enteral nutrition
- Dose: Demand-orientated, 2–3 doses/day

6. Oxycodone slow release
- Indication: Basic analgesia, WHO level III
- Route: po
- Dose: Demand-orientated, 2–3 doses/day

7. Fentanyl-TDS (patch)
- Indication: Basic analgesia, WHO level III; where the enteral route is unavailable
- Route: Transdermal
- Dose: Demand-orientated, change of patches every 2–3 days

8. Buprenorphine-TDS (patch)
- Indication: Basic analgesia, WHO level III; where the enteral route is unavailable
- Route: Transdermal
- Dose: Demand-orientated, change of patches every 3–7 days

Caveat: Where slow release and immediate release analgesics are combined, the combination of WHO level II and level III drugs should be avoided.

Supplemental Medication

Tilidine drops
- Indication: Breakthrough pain, WHO level II
- Route: po
- Dose: Around 50% of regular dose, PRN every 3–4 hours

Tramadol drops/capsules

- Indication: Breakthrough pain, WHO level II
- Route: po
- Dose: Around 50% of regular dose, PRN every 3–4 hours

Morphine sulphate tablets fast release

- Indication: Breakthrough pain, WHO level III
- Route: po
- Dose: Around 50% of regular dose, PRN every 3–4 hours

Morphine sulphate elixir/drops

- Indication: Breakthrough pain, WHO level III
- Route: po
- Dose: Around 50% of regular dose, PRN every 3–4 hours

Fentanyl citrate transmucosal (OTFC, "Lollipops")

- Indication: Breakthrough pain, WHO level III
- Route: po/trans mucosal
- Dose: See drug information sheet

Buprenorphine sublingual tablets

- Indication: Breakthrough pain, WHO level III
- Route: sublingual
- Dose: See drug information sheet

PCA pumps

- Indication: Basic analgesia, problems with enteral route of administration or resorption
- Route: iv (via CVC, Port, etc.), sc
- Dose: Demand-orientated, PCA function with or without continuous background infusion

Opioid Therapy-Management of Side Effects and Complications

Respiratory Depression

Pain is the physiological antagonist of opioid-induced respiratory depression. Therefore, opioids should be titrated slowly according to the pain intensity. Respiratory depression is most likely with high opioid peak serum concentrations and can be avoided by slow administration. A common problem is the deteriorating vigilance of patients with progressing cancer, which adds to opioid-induced sedation. This should not lead to a dose reduction or cease of opioid therapy with increasing pain intensity in pre-terminal patients.

Naloxone:

- Opioid-induced respiratory depression
- Dose: Titration of doses of 0.04 mg iv until respiratory depression resolves; beware of rebound narcosis

Constipation

- Lactulose
  Dose: 2–3 times daily as required
- Coloxyl and Senna
  Dose: 1–2 tablets BD
- Macrogol
  Dose: Once or twice daily

Nausea and Vomiting

- Haloperidol (1st line)
  Dose: 3 × 5 drops po or via feeding tube
- Metoclopramide (2nd line)
  Dose: 3 × 10–20 drops po or via feeding tube

- Ondansetron (3rd line)
  Dose: 1–2 × 4–8 mg po or iv

Pruritus

Opioid rotation

Therapy with Adjuvant Drugs

- Amitriptyline
  For burning-type neuropathic pain
  Dose: 25–75 mg po/day
- Duloxetine
  Dose: 20–60 mg po/day
- Gabapentin
  For neuropathic pain
  Dose: 300–3600 mg po/day
- Pregabalin
  Dose: 150–600 mg po/day
- Dexamethasone
  For pain related to capsular tension of parenchymal organs (caused by edema or metastasis), nerve compression caused by tumor or metastasis
  Dose: Start with 32 mg po or iv, then decrease dose until reaching a dose of 4 mg po or iv/day

Interventional Pain Therapy

Neurolytic techniques

Neurolytic techniques should only be used as a last line treatment, for example with pancreatic carcinoma (neurolysis of the coeliac plexus) or pelvic tumors (intrathecal neurolysis).

Spinal or Epidural Catheters

The advantage of spinal or epidural catheters is that they may allow a reduction in opioid dose compared to oral or parenteral administration.

The disadvantage is the high personal and technical expenditure and the risk of technical complications or malfunction.

Psychological Therapy

- Emotional and practical support and advice, pain coping strategies, crisis intervention, treatment of any associated depression
- Support of relatives/caregivers
- Pain control strategies:
  Relaxation and imagination techniques, stress management

Bibliography

Bruera E, Portenoy RK (2003) Cancer pain: assessment and management. Cambridge University Press, Cambridge

Fallon M, Hanks G, Cherny N (2006) Principles of control of cancer pain. BMJ 332:1022–1024

Fisch MJ, Burton AW (2007) Cancer pain management. McGraw-Hill Medical, New York

Rozen D, Grass GW (2005) Perioperative and intraoperative pain and anesthetic care of the chronic pain and cancer pain patient receiving chronic opioid therapy. Pain Pract 5:18–32

6 Postoperative Pain

M. Schenk, T. Machholz, S.A. Schug, G. Jaehnichen, S.J. Harper

Interventional pain therapeutic procedures must be done with the informed consent of the patient. The choice of a specific pain therapeutic treatment depends primarily on the site and type of surgery performed. There may be indications or contraindications pertaining to the patient's co-morbidity and prior medications, as well as to the surgery itself. The patient's preferences should always be taken into account. Information about the procedure and risks of a planned pain therapeutic treatment should be discussed with the patient during the preoperative anesthetic assessment and should be documented on the anesthetic record.

On the basis of agreements between surgical and anesthetic bodies, we can differentiate between four different organizational models of postoperative pain therapy:

1. Anesthetic consultation for a single pain problem
2. Management of selected pain therapeutic measures through the anesthetist or an established acute pain service (APS)
3. Transfer of the complete postoperative pain management to the anesthetist or an acute pain service
4. Interdisciplinary pain service

In our clinic, the organizational model 2 is implemented, combined with anesthetic consultations for single pain problems (model 1).

Pain therapy through nursing staff (nurse controlled analgesia, NCA) is performed on the wards by nurses following orders from physicians or the anesthetist who gave the anesthetic.

The Acute Pain Service (APS) is organized by the Department of Anesthesia and Intensive Care Medicine, and is responsible for patients who are managed using the following postoperative analgesic techniques 2–4:

1. Nurse Controlled Analgesia (NCA)
2. Patient Controlled Analgesia (PCA)
3. Epidural Analgesia (EDA)
4. Other Catheter Techniques

On weekdays, the APS consists of a doctor and a nurse from the pain medicine center. On nights and weekends a dedicated anesthetist is assigned to the pain service to manage APS patients. If the "pain service" anesthetist is occupied with other work, the senior anesthetist on call is informed immediately to organize or take over the Acute Pain Service. Thus, continuous care for all pain patients can be achieved. All APS team members carry a pager so that they can be immediately contacted.

On weekdays, the doctor responsible for the APS performs daily ward rounds to assure a high quality of postoperative pain treatment and to document the performed measures. During these ward rounds problems may be discussed with the responsible physicians and nurses. On weekends and public holidays, the ward rounds are performed by the "pain service" anesthetist.

6.1 Nursing Staff-Managed Pain Therapy (Nurse Controlled Analgesia, NCA)

NCA is a method of systemic drug administration. On the basis of the WHO Guidelines for treatment of cancer pain, non-opioid analgesics (paracetamol, NSAIDS and cox-II inhibitors), as well as opioids (morphine, fentanyl, tramadol) can be used.

Administration of drugs is performed by the nursing staff following standing orders or a special order of a physician.

Indication

- NCA is especially used in children or in cognitively impaired patients, who are unable to handle PCA or have no other form of pain therapy
- NCA is also indicated in any other surgical patient who for any other reason has no PCA or catheter technique for pain therapy

Procedure

- NCA should start directly after surgery in the recovery room. Pain intensity should be measured with a visual analogue scale (VAS) and documented by the recovery room staff. Based on this score, pain medicine can be given (standing orders, orders by the anesthetist)

Non-Opioid Analgesics

Paracetamol

- Adults: 1 g oral/rectal (4–6-hourly) or 1 g iv (Perfalgan)
- Schoolchildren: 500 mg oral/rectal or 500 mg IV
- Toddlers: 250 mg rectal
- Infants: 125 mg rectal

(General dose formula for single dose: 20 mg/kg body weight)

Non-Steroidal Anti-Inflammatory Drugs (NSAIDS)

- Diclofenac: 3 × 50 mg rectal

Cox-II Inhibitors

- Parecoxib: 2 × doses 40 mg iv

Opioids

- Fentanyl: 30–50 mg bolus iv, repeated every 3 minutes until patient comfortable

- Morphine: 1–3 mg bolus iv, repeated every 3 minutes until patient comfortable
- Tramadol: 50 mg bolus iv, repeated every 3 minutes until patient comfortable

Complications

- Incompatibility and allergic reactions to administered drugs (especially non-opioid analgesics)
- Overdose, especially of opioids

Management of Complications

- Signs of incompatibility or allergic reaction should prompt an immediate halt of drug administration. In case of an allergic reaction, appropriate measures should be taken as per Advanced Life Support guidelines (oxygen, adrenaline, etc.) according to the severity of the allergic reaction
- In case of a suspected opioid overdose, patient's level of consciousness, ventilation, blood pressure and heart rate must be monitored continuously. Depending on the severity of symptoms, naloxone should be considered
- The physician in charge of the patient must be informed

Documentation

Pain intensity (VAS) together with blood pressure, heart-rate and ventilation rate should be determined by the nursing staff on a regular basis (at least once hourly) and documented on the anesthetic record, together with the analgesics administered to the patient.

Quality Control

Quality control of NCA is performed by the staff on the surgical wards through documentation of pain intensity and analgesic administration in the patient's chart. This allows the patient's team and/or the APS to check the pain control during ward rounds.

6.2 Patient Controlled Analgesia (PCA)

PCA is a form of systemic administration of analgesics. It allows the patient to control the rate of iv administration of an analgesic drug herself thereby providing feedback control. To achieve a satisfactory pain control, the patient must be sufficiently educated about the handling of the PCA pump.

Technical Issues

For PCA, only specially designed PCA pumps should be used (Manufacturers: Vygon, Smith, Graseby, Hospira). Pumps of different manufacturers differ in technical details: some pumps work using a hydraulic system others are electronic and can be programmed. Pumps can be powered by electricity or battery.

Preparation of the PCA pumps with different analgesics:

Fentanyl:

- Concentration: 50 mcg/ml
- Bolus dose: 20 mcg
- Lockout interval: 5 min
- No 4-hour dose limit and no continuous background infusion

Morphine:

- Concentration: 2 mg/ml
- Bolus dose: 1 mg
- Lockout interval: 5 min
- No 4-hour dose limit and no continuous background infusion

Tramadol:

- Concentration: 10 mg/ml
- Bolus dose: 20 mg
- Lockout interval: 5 min
- No 4-hour dose limit and no continuous background infusion

Indications

The majority of surgical procedures in general surgery, orthopedic surgery, heart surgery, obstetrics, urology, maxillo facial surgery and ENT surgery are a potential indication for pain therapy via PCA.

Patients suitable for PCA should meet the following criteria:

- Patients should be intellectually and physically able to handle the PCA pump
- Patients should be able to assess their pain intensity using the VAS
- Caution, but not a contraindication, in patients who abuse alcohol or drugs
- Severe impairment of liver function, renal function, heart and CNS must be excluded
- Caution in the presence of sleep apnea

Procedure

Postoperative pain therapy with PCA can be started in the recovery room or on the ward.

PCA Start in the Recovery Room

Immediately after the patient arrives from surgery, pain intensity should be determined and, according to the intensity, analgesics should be administered (after standing order, individual order). Before connecting the patient to the PCA, he should be pain-free or with a low pain intensity.

The indication for a PCA should be revised by the anesthetist responsible for the patient, and if the PCA is used the patient should (again) be instructed in the handling of the PCA pump. During his stay in the recovery room, the patient's vital parameters and pain intensity should be determined (at least every 10 minutes) and documented on the patient's chart.

Before discharge to the ward, the pain service should be informed about the patient, and his details should be given (name, ward, type of surgery, current pain therapy, pain intensity and possible complications). A PCA protocol should be started, showing the start time of the PCA, type of the analgesic drug, drug concentration and the name of the ordering anesthetist.

PCA Started on the Ward

If a patient scheduled for a PCA does not get one in the recovery room (no pain, too drowsy, no PCA-pump available, etc.) the pain service must be informed before the patient is discharged to the ward.

In this case, the pain service can review the patient on the ward, and if necessary supply a PCA pump after documentation of pain intensity, blood pressure, pulse and respiratory rate. The pain service must ensure that the patient is able to use the PCA without problems.

Safety

- An infusion must run alongside the PCA pump at all times. The giving set of the infusion must have an anti-reflux valve to prevent

backflow of analgesic drug from the PCA into the infusion and an anti-syphon valve.
- Administration of additional opioid analgesics or sedatives is contraindicated, if not checked with the pain service
- The ward nurses are responsible for monitoring the patient. There should be hourly monitoring and documentation of vital parameters for the first 4 hours after starting the PCA
- All drugs and equipment necessary for resuscitation must be on wards where PCA pumps are used
- Due to the possibility of opioid-induced constipation, prophylactic measures for bowel stimulation (in agreement with the surgeon) must be undertaken if the PCA pump is in use for more than 24 hours

Complications

- Incompatibility and allergic reactions
- Drug overdose with possible severe complications caused by:
  - Use of the PCA pump by anyone other than the patient
  - Wrong handling of the PCA pump by the patient
  - Analgesic drug in the giving set leading to unintended boluses
  - Programming or dilution error

Management of Complications

- In case of life-threatening complications, resuscitation must be started immediately as per Advanced Life Support guidelines. The hospital resuscitation team must be informed. Complications due to opioid overdose should be treated with naloxone iv
- In case of non-urgent complications, the APS should be informed via pager or telephone

Documentation

- A PCA protocol especially designed for PCA should be used.
- In the recovery room vital parameters, pain intensity and the PCA pump setting should be determined and documented on the PCA protocol every 30 minutes
- During the first four hours the PCA is running, vital signs and side effects should be documented every hour
- After the first four hours the PCA is in use, documentation of the necessary parameters can be performed every two hours. If the patient is asleep at night, waking him up to determine pain intensity is not necessary but vital signs must still be measured and documented
- The PCA protocol and the patient's chart should be with the patient at all times

Quality Control

The APS visits all PCA patients at least once a day. During this visit, efficacy of the analgesic therapy and possible side effects should be determined and documented on the PCA protocol. These protocols should be analyzed for quality control from time to time.

6.3 Epidural Analgesia (EDA)

This type of regional analgesia for postoperative pain therapy is performed via insertion of an epidural catheter usually before the operation. Informed consent with the usual documentation is necessary before the procedure.

In a majority of patients, administration of analgesic drugs via the catheter is performed on a continuous basis with a syringe driver or in fusion pump. The analgesics of choice are usually the local anesthetic Ropivacaine 0.1–0.2% together with Sufentanil 0.5 µg/ml or Fentanyl 1–2 µg/ml.

Technical aspects

For drug administration, syringe drivers and infusion pumps from different companies are used (Abbott, Braun, Deltec, Fresenius, IVAC, SIMS). Patient controlled techniques are preferred to continuous infusion alone.

Indications

Patients suitable for EDA for postoperative analgesia should meet the following criteria:

- They should be able to assess their pain intensity using the VAS
- Caution in coexisting abuse of alcohol, medicine or drugs
- Severe impairment of liver function, renal function, heart and CNS must be excluded (relative contraindication)

Before catheter insertion, the following conditions should be excluded:

- Coagulopathy
- Allergic reactions to local anesthetics
- Severe impairment of liver or renal function and heart or blood pressure (relative contraindication)
- CNS disorders (neuromuscular disorders and peripheral nerve lesions)
- Acute spinal disorders
- Degenerative spinal disorders, especially in the presence of radicular deficits

- Where there are acute neurological deficits, for medico-legal reasons the technique should be avoided. If it is felt to be in the patient's best interests, a formal detailed neurologic examination should be performed and documented prior to the procedure being undertaken
- Septic conditions or local infection of the puncture site

As an alternative to continuous epidural analgesia, PCA may be used.

Provision of Epidural Analgesia

Pain intensity, vital parameters and catheter position should be determined and documented in the recovery room. The catheter should then be connected to the infusion pump or syringe driver. To exclude spinal catheter placement, 3 ml plain Bupivacaine 0.5% (or an equivalent amount of another local anaesthetic) can be injected as a test dose.

After confirmation of correct catheter placement, boluses of 5ml Bupivacaine 0.5% or ropivacaine 0.75% are given. Epidural catheters inserted as part of a CSE procedure should be tested particularly stringently. Block height can be determined using ice, pin prick or cold spray.

The initial continuous infusion rate is between 5 and 10 ml/h. In case of insufficient analgesia it can be increased to a maximum of 16 ml/h (be vigilant for local anesthetic toxicity or impaired ventilation if opioids are used additionally). If patient controlled epidural analgesia is used, a bolus of 2–4 ml with a lockout time of 20–30 min should be programmed.

Patients should not be sent to the ward without clear instructions about the infusion rate and a prepared local anesthetic/opioid solution in a syringe or bag.

Pain intensity, analgesic spread and vital parameters are documented at defined intervals. Before discharge to the ward, the APS needs to be informed to take over the pain management of the patient.

Ongoing Management:

Acute Pain Service Responsibilities

- All changes of the infusion rate or single bolus injections
- Daily ward rounds and quality control
- Daily check of the catheter insertion site
- Dressing changes
- Dose reduction/weaning
- Cessation of the infusion therapy and catheter removal

Ward Staff Responsibilities:

- Patient monitoring
- Documentation of monitored parameters
- Changing syringes or bags of local anesthetics

Safety

- Administration of additional analgesics or sedatives must be checked with the pain service
- Administration of benzodiazepines is contraindicated
- APS must be informed in case of insufficient analgesia, side effects, complications related to the pain therapy or a developing infection

Conditions for Epidural Catheter Removal

- The timing of removal with regard to thrombembolic prophylaxis should follow established international guidelines
- Pain-free interval without analgesic infusion at least 8 h

Complications

- Allergic reaction or intolerance
- Neurological complications
  Reasons for neurological complications:
- Secondary perforation of the dura (catheter migration)
- Development of an epidural hematoma
- Development of an epidural infection
- Respiratory depression secondary to epidural opioids (Sufentanil, Fentanyl). The treatment is as for opioid-induced respiratory depression via any route (naloxone iv but NB opioid rebound)

Management of Complications

- In case of insufficient analgesia, the APS should be informed immediately
- If vital parameters are impaired, the APS or the resuscitation team must be informed, according to the severity of the situation
- In case of neurological dysfunction the APS as well as a neurologist should be consulted immediately

Documentation

Clinical parameters (level of consciousness, blood pressure, heart rate check of sensory and motor function of the legs) should be documented after starting the analgesic infusion or after changes of the infusion rat in 1 hour intervals for the first 4 hours. The parameters are documented on the APS chart. After bolus injection, monitoring of blood pressur and heart rate is necessary for a period of at least 30 minutes.

Quality Control

See "PCA Pumps".

6.4 Continuous Peripheral Nerve Analgesia

This type of regional analgesia for postoperative pain therapy is performed via insertion of a catheter, usually before the operation. Informed consent with the usual documentation is necessary before the procedure.

In the majority of patients the analgesic drug is delivered continuously using a syringe driver or infusion pump. The analgesic of choice is usually the local anesthetic ropivacaine 0.2%

Technical Aspects

For drug administration, syringe drivers and infusion pumps from various manufacturers are used (Abbott, Braun, Fresenius, IVAC, SIMS). Patient controlled techniques are preferred over continuous infusion alone.

Indications

Patients suitable for continuous peripheral regional analgesia should meet the following criteria:

- They should be able to assess their pain intensity using a VAS
- Severe impairment of liver function, renal function, heart and CNS must be excluded (relative contraindication)

Before catheter insertion, the following conditions should be excluded:

- Coagulopathy
- Allergic reactions to local anesthetics
- Severe impairment of liver or renal function and heart function or blood pressure (relative contraindication)
- CNS disorders (neuromuscular disorders and peripheral nerve lesions)
- Acute spinal disorders
- In case of acute neurologic deficits, for medico-legal reasons the technique should be avoided. If for any reason it is used, a neurologic examination should be performed and documented
- Septic conditions or local infections of the puncture site

Procedure

Pain intensity and vital parameters are determined and documented in the recovery room. Correct catheter placement should have been checked by the anesthetist at the end of surgery, and should be rechecked in recovery before connecting the catheter to a syringe driver/infusion pump.

If the catheter is in the right position, local anesthetic boluses of a total dose of 10–30 ml are applied. Testing of anesthetic spread should be performed with ice, cold spray or a pinprick test.

The initial continuous infusion rate is between 6–14 ml/h. In case of insufficient analgesia it can be increased to a maximum of 16 ml/h (caveat: local anesthetic toxicity). If patient controlled analgesia is used, a bolus of 4 ml with a lockout time of 30 min should be programmed.

Patients should not be sent to the ward without clear instruction about the infusion rate and without a prepared local anesthesia solution in a syringe or bag.

Pain intensity, analgesic spread and vital parameters are documented on the pain service record at defined intervals. Before discharge to the ward, the APS needs to be informed to take over the pain management of the patient.

Acute Pain Service Responsibilities

- All changes of the infusion rate or single bolus injections
- Daily ward rounds and quality control
- Daily check of the catheter insertion site
- Dressing changes
- Dose reduction
- Cessation of the infusion therapy and catheter removal

Ward Responsibilities

- Patient monitoring
- Documentation of monitored parameters
- Change of syringes or bags with the local anesthetic

Safety

The APS must be informed in case of insufficient analgesia, side effects, complications in connection with the pain therapy (neurologic symptoms) or development of an infection.

Conditions for Catheter Removal

1. No acute bleeding disorder
2. The time after the last heparin administration with low-dose/high-dose heparin should be 4 hours, and with aspirin it should be 2 days
3. The pain-free interval without analgesic infusion should be at least 8 h

Point 2 only applies for peripheral catheters in regions where external compression in case of bleeding is not possible.

Complications

- Allergic reaction or intolerance of local anesthetics
- Neurological complications
  Reasons for neurological complications are:
- Development of hematoma
- Development of infection

Management of Complications

In case of insufficient analgesia, the APS should be informed immediately. If vital parameters are impaired, the APS or the resuscitation team must be informed according to the severity of the situation. In case of neurological dysfunction the APS and a neurologist should be consulted.

Documentation

Clinical parameters (blood pressure, heart rate, check of sensory and motor function) should be documented after start of the analgesic infusion or after changing the infusion rate in 1 hour intervals for the first 4 hours. The parameters are documented on the APS chart. After bolus injection monitoring of blood pressure and heart rate is necessary for a period of at least 30 minutes.

Quality Control

See "PCA Pumps".

6.5 Systemic Analgesia

IV, PCA, epidural analgesia and continuous peripheral nerve analgesia can be supplemented with non-opioid analgesics. With this measure, analgesia can be improved and an opioid-sparing effect can be achieved.

Non-Opioid Analgesia: Preoperative Administration

- Celecoxib
  Dose: 100–200 mg po
- Parecoxib
  Dose: 40 mg iv
- Paracetamol
  Dose 1 g iv
- Metamizol
  Dose 1 g iv

Non-Opioid Analgesia: Intraoperative Administration

- Parecoxib
  Dose: 40 mg iv
- Paracetamol
  Dose: 1 g iv
- Metamizol
  Dose 1–2 g iv

Non-Opioid Analgesia: Postoperative Administration

- Parecoxib
  Dose 2 × 40 mg iv (12 hourly)

- Paracetamol
  Dose 1g iv (6 hourly)
- Metamizol
  Dose 1g iv (4 hourly)

NSAIDS and Cox–II inhibitors impair renal function and can lead to acute renal failure in predisposed patients. Predisposing factors include existing renal impairment and dehydration. Intraoperative factors are large volume shifts with the risk of hypovolaemia. IV non-opioid analgesics should only be used in normovolemic patients without the risk of major bleeding.

NSAIDS and Cox–II inhibitors should not be given to patients with renal impairment or suspected large intraoperative volume shifts.

Bibliography

American Society of Anesthesiologists Task Force on Acute Pain Management (2004) Practice guidelines for acute pain management in the perioperative setting: an updated report by the American Society of Anesthesiologists Task Force on Acute Pain Management. Anesthesiology 100:1573–1581

Australian and New Zealand College of Anesthetists, Faculty of Pain Medicine (2005) Acute pain management: scientific evidence, 2nd edn. Melbourne: Australian and New Zealand College of Anesthetists (available at www.nhmrc.gov.au or www.anzca.edu.au/resources/books-and-publications)

Department of Defense, Veterans Health Administration (2002) Clinical practice guideline for the management of postoperative pain, version 1.2. Department of Defense, Veterans Health Administration, Washington DC (available at www.oqp.med.va.gov)

Institute for Clinical Systems Improvement (2006) Health care guideline: assessment and management of acute pain , 6th edn. ICSI, Bloomington 2006 (available at www.icsi.org)

Rosenquist RW, Rosenberg J (2003) United States Veterans Administration: postoperative pain guidelines. Reg Anesth Pain Med 28:279–288 (guideline material available at www.oqp.med.va.gov)

Rozen D, Grass GW (2005) Perioperative and intraoperative pain and anesthetic care of the chronic pain and cancer pain patient receiving chronic opioid therapy. Pain Pract 5:18–32

Shorten G (2006) Postoperative pain management: an evidence-based guide to practice. Saunders Elsevier, Philadelphia

American Society of Regional Anesthesia and Pain Medicine (ASRA). Second Consensus Statement on Neuraxial Anesthesia and Anticoagulation 2002 (available at http://www.asra.com/consensus-statements/2.html)

Subject Index